IF
FAT , FAT
YOU
AT!

Fasting Frenzy for Ultra-Fast
Fat Loss

A Little Book by:

Paeti Gustav Xaviers

This book is dedicated to all of
those fellow people who
have struggled with fat loss,
seemingly without hope,
just like me.

Introduction:

I was a chubby kid. As a teen, I constantly struggled in an effort to become reasonably and decently not so "pleasingly" plump. In my twenties, I kind of gave up hope and wore plus sizes. Then, in my early thirties, I concocted a diet that WORKED. I lost up to 2 pounds a day (2 pounds per day was the norm) and, it seemed, instantly I was wearing a junior size 5 and finally had FUN buying a new wardrobe.

If this sounds like you, or you are just one of those people who wants or needs to lose weight ultra-fast (including fat), give this diet a try. It's the ONLY diet that EVER worked for me, consistently, every time life's living found me on the weight gained path.

In addition to ultra-fast fat loss, I was able to keep the weight OFF for 10 years, without re-fasting, by eating a "normal" (one little on the hefty size) meal per day, usually around 4:00 p.m. But, whenever you eat, try not to eat later than 3 hours before bedtime.

***

REMEMBER: Get in touch with your health practitioner

before embarking critically on this or any weight loss diet.

FAT, FAT YOU AT!

If FAT, FAT you AT, there is a crash fasting fast diet that always and only worked for me. But first, check with your health practitioner to make sure your body can sustain the diet. You can always break the

fasting days up and do
a little at a time (every
other day or so).

As mentioned, I lost
weight FAST! Fat,
included. I fasted for
15 days and lost 30
pounds with the help of
two dieting aids:
DEXATRIM (Max is
recommended) and

GRAPEFRUIT SEED EXTRACT

(NutriBiotic Vegan Capsules, Max strength 250 mg is good) [Products available at Walmart or Walgreens]. You will also need a Potassium Supplement (99 mg) and have Matzos (Manischewitz Brand is

good) on hand
[Products should be
available also at
Walmart or
Walgreens].

In the morning, I would
first take a Dexatrim
and a grapefruit extract
pill. Then I would have
2 cups of light and
sweet coffee (use

Truvia for sweetness
and your favorite flavor
of Coffeemate
[Walmart or
Walgreens]). This
helps get your system
awake and ready to get
going while at the same
time, helping you to
move your bowels.
Morning coffee is
followed by up to 3 tall

glasses of filtered water. Take your time. No need to rush through the coffee and water.

After I felt the urdge to "go" [move my bowels] and relieved myself, I would take my Potassium Supplement.

Then, all day I would drink high caffeine content diet soda (up to 2 2L bottles per day - I drink Pepsi Max [Walmart]), diet iced tea [Lipton Diet Lemmon] and water. If I felt too much bubbly from the soda, I would remove the cap and let it go flat prior to drinking. The flat soda is really the best, but occasional bubbly is refreshing, especially with ice on a warm or hot day.

I would try NOT to eat all day. I had to move SLOWLY to avoid passing out from light-headedness as the days passed. So move SLOWLY. AND DO NOT EXERCISE. But on the days when I absolutely could not go another minute or day without food, I would slowly eat 1 matzo (up to 5 in one day). Then get back to the fasting the next day.

Simple as that. Take all your regular medications. Just be careful about light-headedness, especially upon waking in the morning and do not fast for more than 28 consecutive days.

Weight Loss Chart

Day	Wt.	Day	Wt.

Day	Wt.	Day	Wt.

Day	Wt.	Day	Wt.

Day	Wt.	Day	Wt.

Day	Wt.	Day	Wt.

Day	Wt.	Day	Wt.

Day	Wt.	Day	Wt.

Personal Notes:

Page -28-

www.ingramcontent.com/pod-product-compliance
Lightning Source LLC
Chambersburg PA
CBHW070938290526
45795CB00003B/1063